SMOOTHIES FOR A HEALTHY HEART

CARDIAC VITALITY

MONIK ROJAS

DEDICATION

To you, who have felt the weight of a life affected by the restless beats of a heart that seems unable to find calm, this book is for you. I know what it is like to live with the uncertainty of symptoms, with the fear of each accelerated heartbeat or that inexplicable tiredness that leaves you without strength. I know what it is like to desire a change, to long for a life in which you can breathe deeply without worrying about your health.

This book is made with the hope of offering you a new perspective, a way to take charge of your well-being, to reconnect with your body, your health and your vitality. Each recipe, each piece of advice, has been created with you in mind, so that you can find relief, strength and the peace of mind that you so deserve.

May this journey be the beginning of a life in which your heart once again becomes synonymous with energy and well-being, where every day you can feel stronger, healthier, and, above all, freer.

With all my love and sincere hope that you find new hope for your life in these pages.

INDEX

INTRODUCTION
Welcome to your journey to a healthy heart.

- How Smoothies can benefit your cardiovascular health.
- What will you find in this book?

CHAPTER 1
Understanding Cardiovascular Health

The Heart: Your engine of life
- Anatomy and function of the heart
- How the cardiovascular system works

Symptoms of cardiovascular problems

- Early signs to look out for (fatigue, dizziness, chest tightness)
- More serious symptoms that require urgent medical attention

- Risk Factors for Heart Health
- Hypertension, high cholesterol, and their impact on the heart
- How lifestyle (smoking, diet, sedentary lifestyle) affects cardiovascular health
- Genetic factors and predisposition

How to take care of your heart effectively

- Balanced diet rich in antioxidants, fiber and healthy fats
- The importance of regular physical exercise

Maintain a healthy weight and manage stress
- Get enough sleep to repair and maintain cardiovascular function
- Importance of regular medical check-ups and monitoring of blood pressure and cholesterol.

INTRODUCTION

WELCOME TO YOUR JOURNEY TO A HEALTHY HEART

Welcome to an exciting journey toward a healthier, more vibrant life! This book is designed to be your ideal companion in the quest for a strong and energetic heart. Here you will discover how simple changes in your diet can have a profound impact on your cardiovascular health, and the best part is that you will enjoy every step of the way.

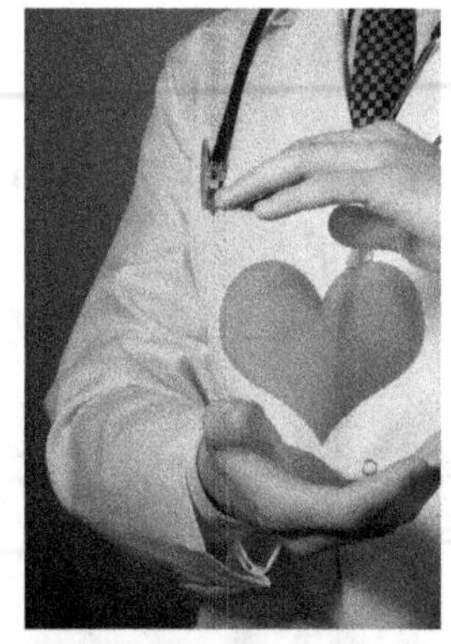

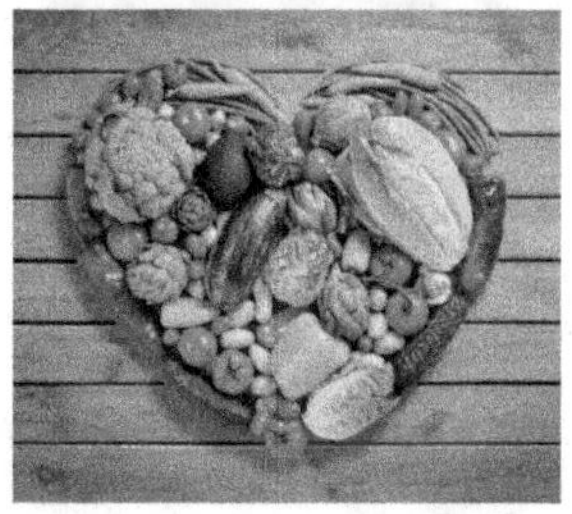

How Smoothies Can Benefit Your Cardiovascular Health

- You may be wondering, how can simple smoothies be so powerful? The answer lies in the ingredients we choose and the way we combine flavors and nutrients to deliver concrete benefits to your heart. Smoothies are a delicious and convenient way to incorporate fruits and vegetables rich in antioxidants, fiber, and healthy fats, all crucial to keeping your cardiovascular system in tip-top shape. Imagine giving your heart a concentrated dose of health with every sip. From lowering blood pressure to improving cholesterol levels, you'll discover how every recipe in this book is designed to effectively support and strengthen your heart.

WHAT WILL YOU FIND IN THIS EBOOK?

In the following pages, we'll guide you through a series of delicious and nutritious recipes, each carefully crafted to maximize the benefits to your heart health. In addition to recipes, we'll provide you with essential information about key ingredients, practical tips for making the most nutritious smoothies, and strategies for integrating these powerful elixirs into your daily life. Get ready to explore how small changes can lead to a big impact on your overall well-being.

So, are you ready to take the first step towards a healthier heart? Let's get started on discovering the power of a smoothie on your cardiovascular health!

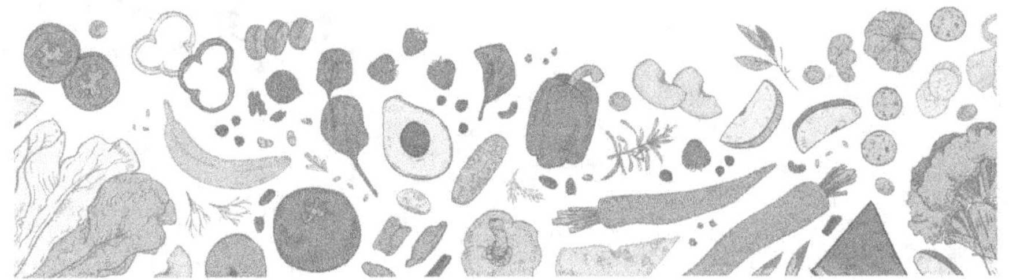

CHAPTER 1

The Heart: Your engine of life.

- Anatomy and function of the heart

The heart is a vital organ that functions as a pump to keep blood moving throughout the body. About the size of a fist, it is located slightly to the left of the chest and is composed primarily of muscle. This heart muscle is special because it can contract continuously and rhythmically without fatigue, allowing the heart to pump blood steadily throughout life.

The heart is divided into four chambers: two atria (upper chambers) and two ventricles (lower chambers). The atria receive blood, while the ventricles pump it. Oxygen-poor blood reaches the right side of the heart and is sent to the lungs to receive oxygen. Oxygen-rich blood then returns to the left side of the heart and is pumped to the rest of the body.

The heart works thanks to a series of valves that ensure that blood flows in the right direction, without backflow. These valves open and close in sync with each heartbeat, controlling blood flow efficiently.

- How the Cardiovascular system works.

The cardiovascular system is made up of the heart, blood vessels (arteries, veins and capillaries) and blood. Its main function is to transport oxygen, nutrients and hormones to the body's cells, as well as removing waste products such as carbon dioxide. The process is as follows:

1. Pulmonary Cycle (Minor Circulation): Deoxygenated blood enters the heart through the vena cava (superior and inferior) into the right atrium. From there, it passes into the right ventricle, which pumps it to the lungs through the pulmonary arteries. In the lungs, the blood receives oxygen and carbon dioxide is released.
2. Systemic Cycle (Major Circulation): Oxygenated blood returns to the heart through the pulmonary veins to the left atrium. It then passes into the left ventricle, which is the strongest chamber of the heart, and from there it is pumped to the entire body through the aorta.

This pumping process is repeated 60 to 100 times per minute, creating the heartbeat. Each beat ensures that oxygen and nutrients reach the body's cells and that waste is removed efficiently.

In short, the heart is the engine that keeps the body running, delivering the essential fuel for life and ensuring that every cell receives what it needs to maintain energy, health and vitality.

Symptoms of Cardiovascular Problems.

- **Early signs to look out for**

The body often sends subtle signals when the heart is not functioning optimally. Recognizing these signals early can be crucial to preventing more serious problems. Below are some of the most common early symptoms:

- Fatigue: Feeling excessively tired or exhausted for no apparent reason can be a sign that your heart is not pumping enough oxygenated blood to your body. This may be because your heart has to work harder to maintain proper blood flow, causing you to feel weak or fatigued even after performing everyday activities.

- Dizziness or fainting: Experiencing dizziness, lightheadedness, or fainting can be a sign that your heart is not pumping enough blood to your brain. This can occur due to low blood pressure or poor circulation, indicating that something is not working properly in your cardiovascular system.
- Chest pressure: Feeling pressure, tightness or discomfort in the chest is one of the most common early signs of heart problems. This sensation, known as angina, can occur during exercise, stress or even at rest, and is a sign that the heart is not getting enough oxygen.
- Shortness of breath (Dyspnea): Shortness of breath, especially during activities that were once easy, can be a sign of heart failure or problems with the circulatory system. The heart is not pumping efficiently, which causes fluid to build up in the lungs, making it difficult to breathe.
- Palpitations or irregular heartbeat: If you feel like your heart is beating too fast, too slow, or irregularly, it may be a sign of cardiac arrhythmias. These irregularities may be harmless in some cases, but in others, they could indicate more serious problems.

More serious symptoms that require urgent medical attention.

There are symptoms that, when present, require immediate medical attention. These signs could be indicating a serious cardiovascular problem, such as a heart attack or heart failure. If you experience any of the following symptoms, it is essential to seek medical help immediately:

Severe chest pain: Sharp, strong, persistent chest pain is a classic sign of a heart attack. This pain often radiates to the left arm, jaw, or back. Although it can vary in intensity, any chest pain that lasts more than a few minutes or that goes away and comes back should be taken seriously.

- Severe shortness of breath: If shortness of breath gets worse quickly, it may be a sign of heart failure or a heart attack. Rapid fluid buildup in the lungs can make breathing extremely difficult.

- Excessive sweating (Cold sweat): Sweating profusely for no apparent reason, accompanied by other symptoms such as chest pain or dizziness, is a warning sign. Cold sweating is the body's response to an internal emergency, such as a heart attack.

- Nausea or vomiting: Although often associated with other health problems, sudden nausea or vomiting, especially if accompanied by chest pain or shortness of breath, can be a sign of heart problems, especially in women.

- Pain in other parts of the body: A heart attack may not only manifest as chest pain. Some people experience pain in areas such as the arms, neck, jaw, back, or stomach. These pains can be subtle or intense, but they should always be taken seriously.

- Loss of consciousness (fainting): Sudden fainting, especially when accompanied by other cardiac symptoms, is a sign that the heart is not pumping enough blood to the brain. This may be the result of an arrhythmia or a heart attack.

Risk Factors for Heart Health.

- Hypertension and high cholesterol: The impact on the heart Hypertension (high blood pressure) and high cholesterol are two of the most common risk factors that negatively affect heart health. Both can go unnoticed, as they often have no clear symptoms, but their long-term impact is significant.

When blood pressure is consistently high, the heart has to work harder to pump blood. This causes overexertion that, over time, weakens the heart muscle. High blood pressure also damages the arteries, making them stiffer and less elastic, which increases the risk of heart attacks and strokes. Cholesterol is a fatty substance that, in excess, can build up on the walls of the arteries. Over time, this forms plaques that restrict blood flow to the heart and other vital organs. This condition, known as atherosclerosis, increases the risk of heart attacks and other serious cardiovascular problems. Both conditions can be controlled and improved through lifestyle changes, such as a balanced diet, regular exercise, and, in some cases, with medications prescribed by a doctor.

Lifestyle: Habits that affect Cardiovascular Health.

Many of the choices we make on a daily basis have a direct impact on our heart health. Lifestyle factors are modifiable, meaning that with the right changes, it is possible to significantly reduce the risk of heart disease. Some of the habits that negatively affect the heart include:

- Smoking: Tobacco is one of the heart's biggest enemies. Smoking damages the walls of your arteries, making it easier for plaque to build up and hardening blood vessels. This increases blood pressure and decreases oxygen levels in the blood, forcing your heart to work harder than necessary. Quitting smoking is one of the best things you can do for your heart health.

- Unhealthy diet: Excessive consumption of foods high in saturated fats, sugars and sodium contributes to increased cholesterol and blood pressure. A diet low in fruits, vegetables, whole grains and healthy fats deprives the heart of the nutrients it needs to function properly. Opting for fresh and natural foods is key to protecting your heart.

- Sedentary lifestyle: Lack of physical activity is closely linked to an increased risk of heart disease. Regular exercise strengthens the heart, improves circulation and helps maintain a healthy weight. A sedentary lifestyle, on the other hand, contributes to weight gain, hypertension and high cholesterol.

Genetic factors and predisposition.

Although much of our cardiovascular risk is under our control, there are some factors that we cannot change. Genetics play an important role in heart health. If you have a family history of heart disease, your risk of developing similar problems is higher.

- Genetic predisposition: If your parents or grandparents have suffered from hypertension, heart attacks, or high cholesterol, you may be more likely to develop these problems. However, knowing this predisposition allows you to take preventive measures, such as regularly monitoring your blood pressure and cholesterol levels, and making adjustments to your lifestyle.

- Congenital conditions: Some people are born with heart defects or conditions that affect how the heart works. Although these conditions cannot be prevented, they can be properly managed with early medical treatment and a healthy lifestyle.

How to take care of your heart effectively.

Taking care of your heart is essential to living a long and healthy life. Below are some key strategies to effectively maintain cardiovascular health.

- Balanced diet: Rich in antioxidants, fiber and healthy fats: A proper diet is essential to keep the heart in optimal condition. Foods rich in antioxidants, fiber and healthy fats help reduce the risk of heart disease.
- Antioxidants: These compounds protect cells from damage caused by free radicals. You can find them in brightly colored fruits and vegetables like berries, spinach, carrots, and tomatoes.
- Fiber: Soluble fiber, present in foods such as oats, legumes and fruits, helps reduce bad cholesterol (LDL) levels in the blood, preventing plaque buildup in the arteries.
- Healthy fats: Incorporating unsaturated fats, such as those found in avocado, nuts, olive oil and fatty fish (salmon, tuna), helps keep cholesterol in balance and protects the arteries.

The importance of regular physical exercise.

Regular exercise is one of the best ways to take care of your heart. Physical activity strengthens the heart muscle, improves circulation and reduces risk factors such as high blood pressure and cholesterol.

Benefits of exercise: Aerobic activities such as walking, running, swimming or cycling improve cardiovascular health. In addition, regular exercise helps maintain a healthy weight and reduces stress, another risk factor for heart disease.

Frequency: At least 150 minutes of moderate physical activity per week is recommended. You can divide this into 30-minute sessions per day, 5 times per week.

Maintain a healthy weight and manage stress.

A healthy weight reduces the workload on the heart and reduces the risk of developing diseases such as hypertension and diabetes, which can damage the cardiovascular system.

- Weight control: To maintain a healthy weight, it is important to balance caloric intake with daily physical activity. Simple dietary changes, such as reducing portions and choosing fresh foods, can help achieve this goal.

- Stress management: Chronic stress can increase blood pressure and release hormones that negatively affect the heart. Techniques such as meditation, yoga, and deep breathing can help you reduce stress. Finding activities you enjoy and practicing self-care are effective ways to stay calm and protect your heart health.

Get enough sleep to repair and maintain cardiovascular function.

Sleep is essential for overall health and, in particular, for the heart. During sleep, the body repairs tissues and regulates important processes such as blood pressure.

Sleep quantity: It is recommended to sleep between 7 and 9 hours per night. Insufficient or poor quality sleep is linked to an increased risk of hypertension, heart disease and obesity.

Tips to improve sleep: Establishing a regular sleep routine, avoiding caffeine before bed, and creating a proper rest environment can help improve sleep quality, which in turn benefits your cardiovascular health.

Importance of regular medical check-ups and monitoring of blood pressure and cholesterol.

Regular medical check-ups are crucial for preventing heart disease.

- Blood Pressure Monitoring: Hypertension is known as the "silent killer" because it often has no symptoms. Checking your blood pressure regularly allows you to detect problems early and take corrective action.

- Cholesterol Control: Measuring your cholesterol levels helps you identify if you are at risk for atherosclerosis, a condition in which the arteries harden due to plaque buildup.

- Medical checkups: In addition to monitoring blood pressure and cholesterol, it's important to have regular blood tests and heart screenings, especially if you have a family history of heart disease or known risk factors.

CHAPTER 2

In this chapter, we'll explore the ingredients that form the foundation of our heart-healthy smoothies. Each of them not only adds flavor and texture, but also provides essential nutrients that strengthen your cardiovascular system. Here, we break down each group of ingredients and their specific benefits for your heart.

Fruits that benefit the Heart.

- **Berries (Strawberries, Blueberries, Raspberries).**

Berries are an excellent source of antioxidants, especially anthocyanins and flavonoids, which help reduce inflammation and protect cells from oxidative damage. Strawberries are rich in vitamin C, which helps improve arterial health, while blueberries and raspberries contain fiber and phytonutrients that may help lower blood pressure and LDL cholesterol.

- **Apples and Pears.**

Both fruits are loaded with soluble fiber, especially pectin, which helps lower blood cholesterol levels. They are also rich in antioxidants and vitamins that contribute to better cardiovascular health. Apples and pears provide a natural sweet treat without adding refined sugars, thus keeping your heart in shape.

- **Avocados**.

Avocados are an excellent source of healthy monounsaturated fats, which are beneficial for the heart. They also contain potassium, which helps regulate blood pressure, and antioxidants such as lutein and vitamin E, which protect the arteries from oxidative damage.

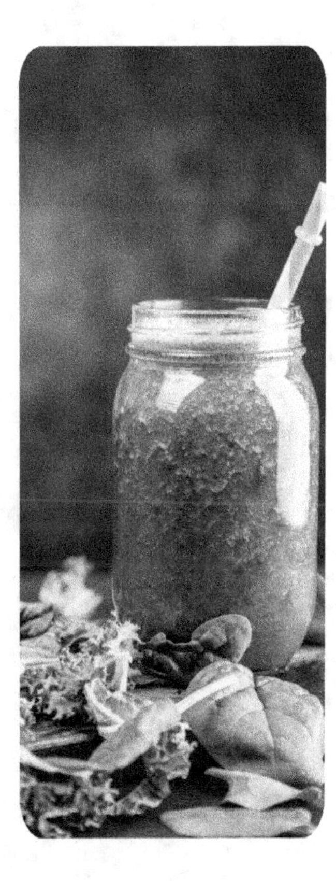

- Spinach

Spinach is rich in nitrates, which can help improve arterial function and reduce blood pressure. It also contains vitamin K, which is essential for cardiovascular health, as well as a variety of antioxidants and minerals.

- Kale (Curly Cabbage)

Kale is a leafy green vegetable that is high in fiber, vitamins A, C, and K, and antioxidants such as flavonoids. These nutrients contribute to heart health by reducing inflammation and improving arterial function.

Seeds and Nuts

- ### *Chia and Flax Seeds.*

These seeds are rich in omega-3 fatty acids, which are essential for keeping the heart healthy. They also contain fiber, which helps control cholesterol levels and maintain digestive health. Chia and flax seeds also provide antioxidants and minerals such as magnesium, which contribute to cardiovascular health.

- ### *Nuts and Almonds*.

Walnuts and almonds are rich in healthy fats, fiber, and antioxidants. Regular consumption of these nuts has been shown to reduce the risk of heart disease by improving HDL (good) cholesterol levels and reducing inflammation.

Healthy Liquids

- ### Almond milk and other alternatives

Almond milk is a low-calorie, cholesterol-free option that can replace cow's milk in your smoothies. It is rich in vitamin E, which acts as an antioxidant to protect your arteries. Other alternatives such as oat milk and hemp milk also offer similar benefits.

- ### *Coconut water*

Coconut water is a natural source of potassium, which helps regulate blood pressure and maintain fluid balance in the body. It is low in calories and can be an effective hydrator, ideal for adding to your smoothies.

Superfoods for the Heart

- **Cocoa Powder**

Unsweetened cocoa powder is rich in flavonoids, which have antioxidant and anti-inflammatory properties. These compounds can help improve circulation and reduce the risk of heart disease.

- **Ginger and Turmeric**

Ginger and turmeric are spices with anti-inflammatory and antioxidant properties. Ginger can help improve circulation and reduce the risk of blood clots, while turmeric contains curcumin, which is known for its positive effects on cardiovascular health.

These ingredients not only add flavor and variety to your smoothies, but they also provide you with the nutrients you need to keep your heart healthy and fit. By combining them in your recipes, you will be taking a big step towards a healthier and more vital life.

CHAPTER 3

Smoothie recipes for cardiovascular health

Welcome to the chapter where we transform healthy ingredients into delicious smoothies that support your cardiovascular health! Each recipe has been crafted to offer specific benefits, from improving your blood pressure to lowering cholesterol. Enjoy these fresh flavors while taking care of your heart.

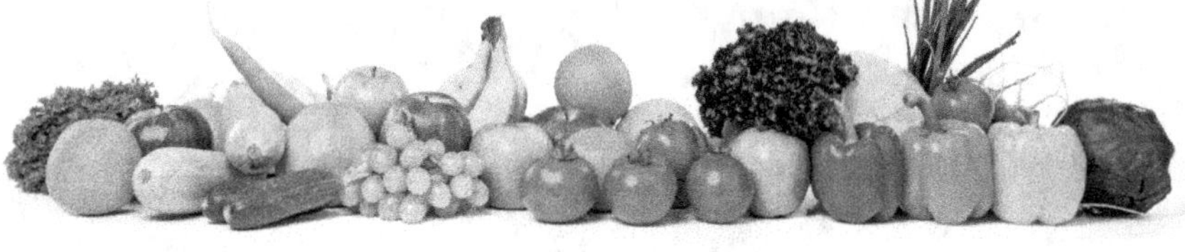

General preparation for all smoothies

- Wash all fresh ingredients thoroughly with plenty of water (fruits and leaves), and make sure they are well drained.
- Peel and cut the fruit into manageable pieces.
- Place all ingredients in the blender, including fruits, vegetables, Greek yogurt, seeds, and any other additives or supplements that the smoothie you have selected contains, along with the base liquid (such as almond milk, coconut water, unsweetened juice, among others).
- Blend at high speed until all ingredients are well mixed and you get a smooth texture.
- Serve immediately in a glass to enjoy its freshness and optimal nutrients.

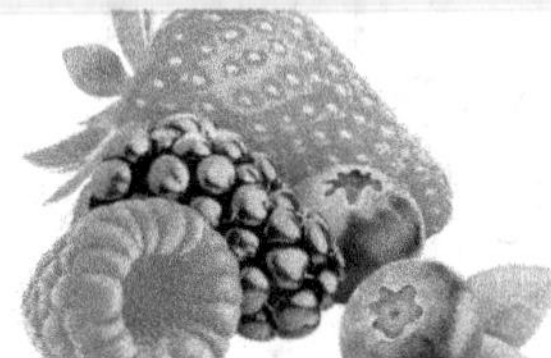
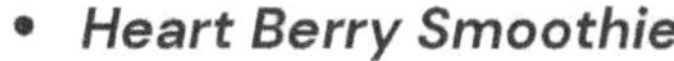

- ***Heart Berry Smoothie***

Benefits: Berries are loaded with antioxidants that help reduce inflammation and protect cells from oxidative damage. They also improve circulation and arterial health.

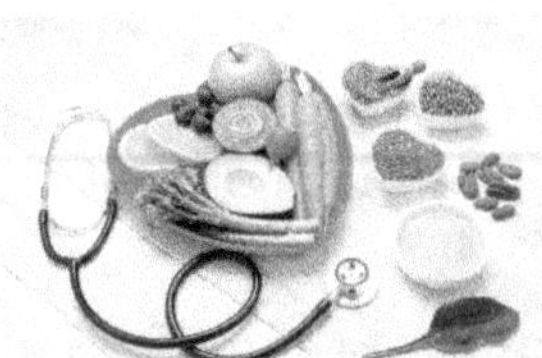

Ingredients:

- 1 cup fresh strawberries
- 1/2 cup blueberries
- 1/2 cup raspberries
- 1 ripe banana or cambur
- 1 cup unsweetened almond milk
- 1 teaspoon honey (optional)

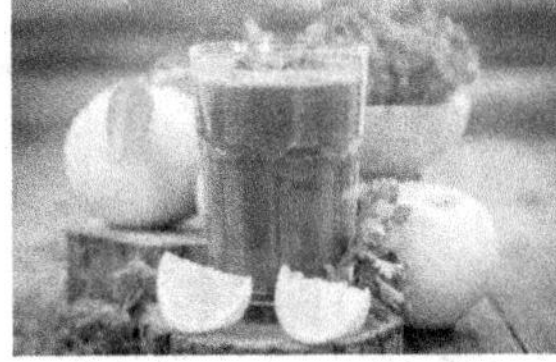

Energizing Green Smoothie.

Benefits: This green smoothie is packed with antioxidants and essential nutrients that help detoxify the body and keep energy high, while supporting heart health.

Ingredients:

1 cup fresh spinach
- 1/2 cup kale
- 1 green apple, cored and cut into pieces
- 1 banana or cambur
- 1 cup coconut water
- Juice of 1 lemon

SMOOTHIES FOR LOWERING CHOLESTEROL

AVOCADO AND SPINACH SMOOTHIE

Benefits: This smoothie combines healthy fats from avocado with nitrates from spinach to help reduce LDL cholesterol and improve arterial health.

Ingredients:

- 1 ripe avocado
- 1 cup fresh spinach
- 1 banana or cambur
- 1 cup unsweetened almond milk
- 1 teaspoon chia seeds

GREEN APPLE AND CINNAMON SMOOTHIE

Benefits: Green apples are rich in fiber that helps reduce cholesterol, while cinnamon provides antioxidant and anti-inflammatory properties.

Ingredients:

- 1 green apple, cored and cut into pieces
- 1/2 teaspoon ground cinnamon
- 1 cup unsweetened almond milk
- 1 teaspoon honey (optional)
- 1/2 cup plain Greek yogurt (optional)

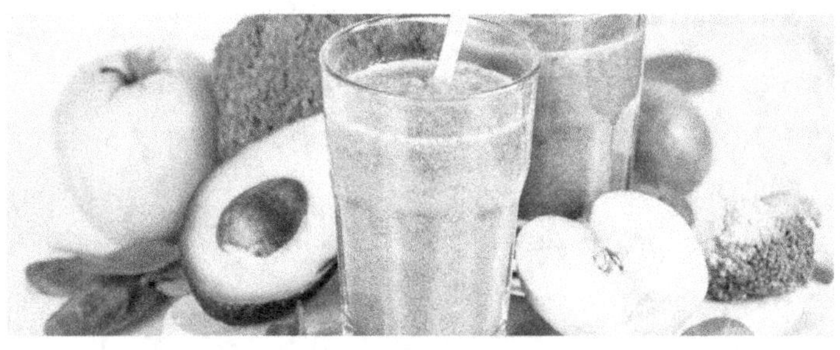

SMOOTHIES FOR HEALTHY BLOOD PRESSURE

Cucumber and Mint Smoothie

Benefits: Cucumber is hydrating and low in sodium, while mint helps improve circulation and digestion, contributing to healthy blood pressure.

Ingredients:

- 1 medium cucumber, peeled and cut into pieces
- 1/4 cup fresh mint leaves
- 1 green apple, cut into pieces
- 1 cup coconut water
- Juice of 1/2 lemon

Beet and Berry Smoothie

Benefits: Beets are rich in nitrates that help reduce blood pressure, while berries provide antioxidants and fiber that improve cardiovascular health.

Ingredients:

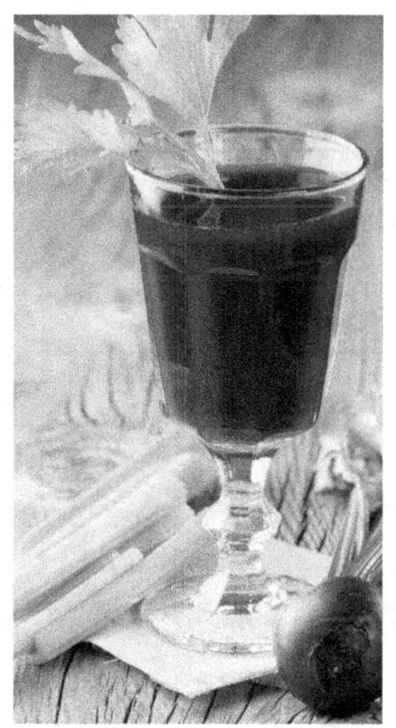

- 1/2 beet cooked and peeled
- 1/2 cup blueberries
- 1/2 cup strawberries
- 1 banana or cambur
- 1 cup unsweetened almond milk.

SMOOTHIES FOR GENERAL HEART HEALTH

Quinoa and Fruit Smoothie

Benefits: Quinoa is a complete source of protein and fiber, while the fruits provide antioxidants and vitamins essential for the heart.

Ingredients:

- 1/2 cup cooked quinoa
- 1 cup strawberries
- 1/2 cup mango
- 1 banana or cambur
- 1 cup unsweetened almond milk

PAPAYA AND CHIA SEED SMOOTHIE

Benefits: Papaya is rich in vitamin C and antioxidants that support heart health, while chia seeds provide omega-3 fatty acids and fiber.

Ingredients:

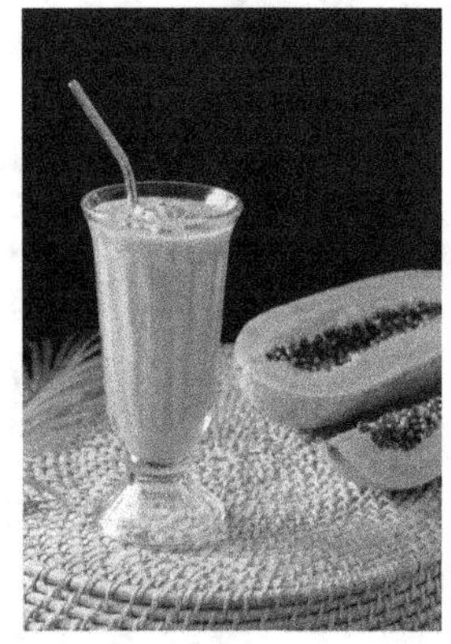

- *1 cup fresh papaya, peeled and cut into pieces*
- *1 tablespoon of chia seeds*
- *1 banana or cambur*
- *1 cup coconut water*

In this chapter, we will offer you practical strategies to integrate smoothies into your daily life and maximize their benefits for cardiovascular health.

7-day plan for a healthy heart.

This 7-day plan is designed to help you introduce smoothies into your diet gradually and effectively, while gaining concrete benefits for your cardiovascular health. Each day has a specific focus to ensure you are getting a variety of essential nutrients for a healthier, stronger heart.

- **Day 1: Antioxidant Smoothies**

Heart Berry Smoothie aims to start your day with a powerful dose of antioxidants. Berries are rich in vitamin C and flavonoids, which helps fight oxidative damage.

- **Day 2: Promoting Arterial Health**

Energizing Green Smoothie, with the goal of including green leafy vegetables to increase nitrates in your diet, which can help improve arterial function and reduce blood pressure.

- **Day 3: Cholesterol Reduction**

Avocado and Spinach Smoothie, with the goal of incorporating healthy fats and fiber to support the reduction of LDL cholesterol and arterial health.

- **Day 4: Blood Pressure Support**

Cucumber and Mint Smoothie, with the aim of using these ingredients to maintain blood pressure at healthy levels and improve hydration.

- **Day 5: Cardiovascular and Digestive Health**

Quinoa and Fruit Smoothie, with the aim of providing complete proteins and fiber for healthy digestion and a strong heart.

- **Day 6: Control Cholesterol and Blood Sugar**

Green Apple and Cinnamon Smoothie, with the aim of using the fiber of the apple and the antioxidant properties of cinnamon to balance blood sugar and reduce cholesterol.

- **Day 7: Superfood Integration**

Papaya and Chia Seed Smoothie, with the aim of maximizing nutrient content, including omega-3 fatty acids and essential vitamins.

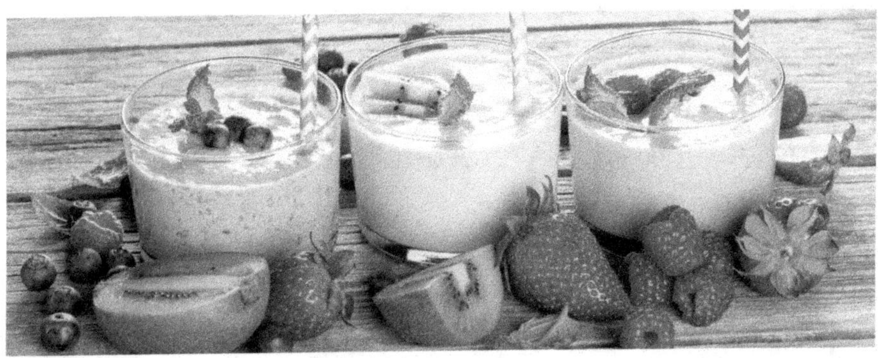

SMOOTHIE CHALLENGE: HOW TO MAKE IT PART OF YOUR ROUTINE?

To get the most out of smoothies and make them an integral part of your life, we propose the following 21-day challenge. This challenge is designed to help you establish sustainable habits and enjoy the benefits in the long term.

Incorporate a smoothie into your daily diet, preferably at breakfast.

- Experimenting and diversifying: Try at least three different recipes during the week to maintain variety and interest.

- Integration and evaluation: Make the smoothie an established part of your daily routine and evaluate the changes in your health.

HOW TO EVALUATE YOUR PROGRESS.

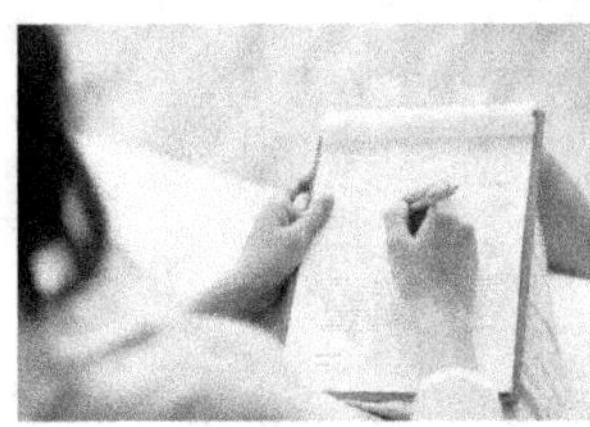

To ensure you're getting the most benefit from your smoothies and staying motivated, it's crucial to evaluate your progress on a regular basis. Here are some effective methods to do so:

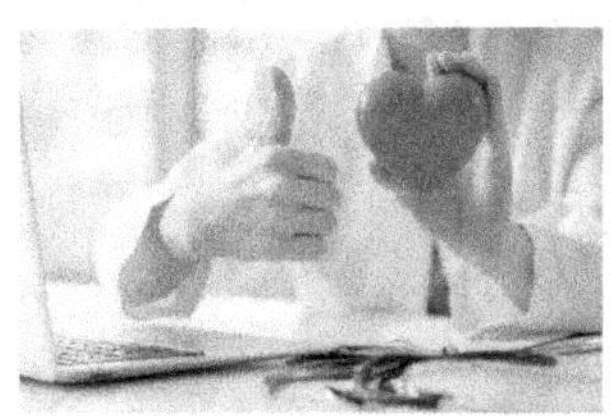

Personal health log. Keep a health journal where you record how you feel each day, changes in your energy, and any improvements in symptoms related to cardiovascular health. Changes in blood pressure, cholesterol levels (if you've had tests), and your general level of well-being.

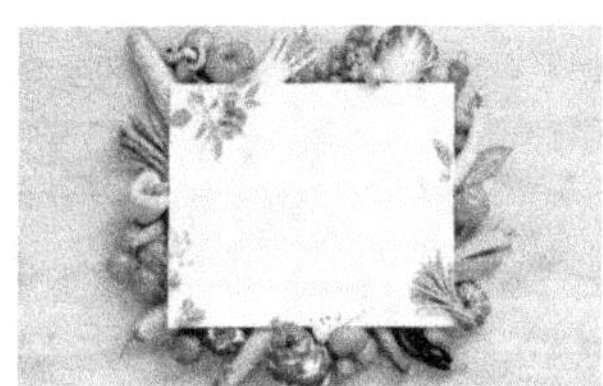

- Habit tracking. Use a food tracking app or spreadsheet to record which smoothies you've consumed and when.
- Goal self-assessment. Review your initial goals and reflect on whether you have achieved them. If you have noticed improvements in your cardiovascular health, how you feel about the changes in your diet, and if the smoothie has become a regular part of your routine.
- Health Check-ups: Schedule regular visits with your health care professional.

CHAPTER 5
CONCLUSIONS

Congratulations on reaching the end of your journey toward better cardiovascular health! In this chapter, we're going to summarize the main benefits of smoothies for your heart and provide you with clear steps to maintain a healthy heart in the long term. We want you to feel inspired and satisfied with everything you've learned, and ready to continue applying this knowledge in your daily life.

Benefits of Smoothies for the Heart

- Powerful Antioxidants: Smoothies that incorporate berries and green vegetables are a rich source of antioxidants. These compounds protect your cells from oxidative damage, reduce inflammation, and promote healthy circulation. By regularly including antioxidant-rich smoothies, you are supporting the health of your arteries and reducing the risk of heart disease.

- Cholesterol Control: Smoothies that combine ingredients like avocado, spinach, and green apple help reduce LDL cholesterol and increase HDL cholesterol. These combinations of healthy fats and fiber not only cleanse your arteries, but also balance your cholesterol levels to keep your heart in optimal condition.

- Blood Pressure Regulation: Smoothies containing cucumber, beetroot, and mint can contribute to healthy blood pressure. These ingredients are loaded with nitrates and potassium, which help relax blood vessels and maintain balanced blood pressure, reducing the risk of hypertension and cardiovascular problems.

- Comprehensive Heart Health Support: By including ingredients like quinoa, papaya, and chia seeds, your smoothies provide a balanced intake of protein, fiber, and healthy fats. These superfoods work together to strengthen your cardiovascular system, improve digestion, and provide long-lasting energy.

Next Steps to Maintain a Healthy Heart

- Continue to integrate smoothies into your routine. You've seen how smoothies can be a powerful tool for improving your cardiovascular health. Continue to make them a regular part of your diet, experimenting with different recipes and adjusting the ingredients to suit your needs and preferences.

- Take a holistic approach to cardiovascular health. Smoothies are just one part of a balanced diet. Combine them with other healthy practices such as a varied diet, regular exercise, and good stress management. This combination will help you maintain a strong and healthy heart in the long run.

- Evaluate and adjust your progress regularly. Consistently assessing your health and well-being will allow you to see the tangible benefits of your efforts. Use a health journal or apps to monitor your progress and make adjustments as needed. Consult with a your healthcare professional will also help you make informed and safe improvements to your diet and lifestyle.

- Inspire others to do the same. Share your experiences and recipes with friends and family to inspire others to improve their cardiovascular health. Mutual motivation and support can make the process more enjoyable and effective for everyone.

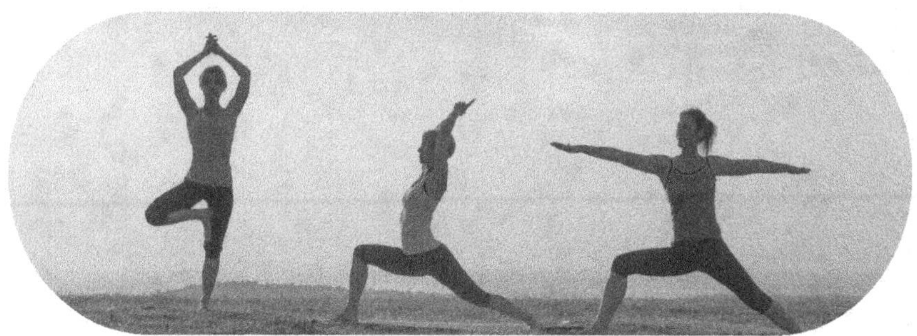

9 798338 794630